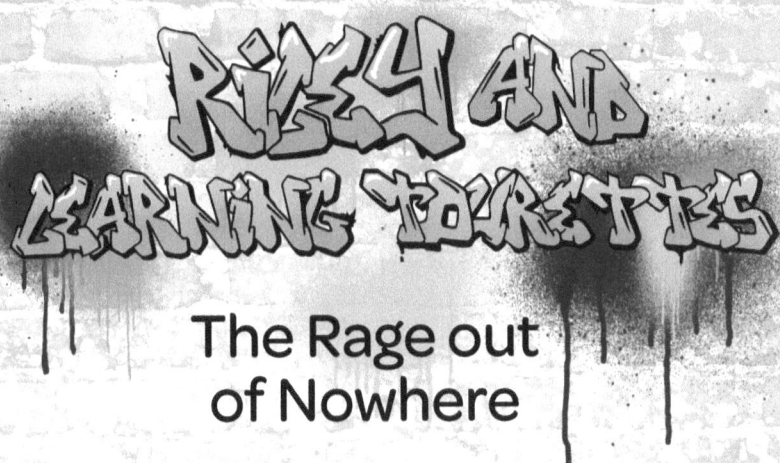

Riley and Learning Tourettes

The Rage out of Nowhere

BOOK ONE

By TM Ritter

FriesenPress
One Printers Way
Altona, MB R0G 0B0
Canada

www.friesenpress.com

First Edition — 2024

ISBN
978-1-03-919733-6 (Hardcover)
978-1-03-919732-9 (Paperback)
978-1-03-919734-3 (eBook)

1. JUVENILE FICTION, HEALTH & DAILY LIVING, DISEASES, ILLNESSES & INJURIES

Distributed to the trade by The Ingram Book Company

Dedication

This book is dedicated to the thousands of families and individuals living with Tourette Syndrome, a very difficult and largely unknown disorder.

In addition, it is dedicated to my husband, Craig, who has stuck it out with me day after day. Through the blunders and mistakes, the triumphs and wins, and the dark days of wanting to give up. For being willing to try new things and listen to me when I suggested new ideas. For being willing to show me grace and love when I was wrong. For being strong enough to admit that you might be wrong too. Thank you for being a true leader in our lives and for every day that you choose to come home and battle through this with us.

For my children, Trey and Brooke, who still love me in spite of all my blunders and mistakes. Who choose every day to keep battling through these tough days. For how strong and brave you both are and oh so stubborn! Don't stop being willing to tackle the hard things of life and show the world just how amazing you are in spite of the wild and wacky things that sometimes go on in your bodies and minds. Believe in the plans and purposes that God has in store for you.

Thank you to the rest of our family and friends that supported us, prayed for us, and did what they could to help us. Thank you to Aimee and Jenny for reading this manuscript over and over and giving me great feedback.

Thank you to Craig's parents, Al and Donna, who have supported us in countless ways through the years.

To my mother, Iris, who is often our greatest support, encourager, and wise counsel. Who led the way for me in demonstrating that even though a parent can make all kinds of mistakes, their child can still turn out OK, and the parent gets better and better too. Thank you for your prayers and guidance. Thank you for your financial support as well.

Lastly, to my aunt Eileen and uncle Greg. Eileen wanted to support us and did financially contribute to this book. Although she and Greg had limited knowledge of what our family experienced, they were always there for us. In the end I wanted badly to have this book published before Eileen passed away, however it was not possible. My hope is that Uncle Greg cherishes this book on her behalf and that somehow she is aware of the difference it makes in others' lives.

Introduction

This story is based on our family's experiences and lives, living with and raising a child diagnosed with Tourette Syndrome. It may be similar to yours or someone you love. It may be different. We entered this journey with our children as we all do: completely naive and beginners. Life has a way of teaching us all what we need to know and then some. It has been a long journey to get to where we are as a family and during the dark days of rages, my husband and I did not think it would ever end. We felt hopeless, lost, desperate, and wanted to give up on many days. You may too.

This story about Riley is intended to demonstrate what those dark days were like for us and our children. It will touch on individual stories of the people around Riley and personal things from Riley himself. Our intention with this story is to bring a hope to those struggling through this time, whether it be the child or the family, friends, and professionals. We have been through this and we were not given any assistance or education as to what was going on with our child. Professionals would try to advise us but they had no training for what was occurring. Their programs did not address what was happening to Riley. It was the hardest thing my husband and I have ever done and our goal is to make it easier for even just one other family.

I, the author and mother, apologize ahead of time for the emotions this story might bring out for you and maybe your child. Every time I read it over again, I cry at certain points. The chapter on Riley's rages is not exaggerated or fabricated in any way. In fact, it leaves a lot of details out. I apologize if it is difficult for the reader; however, a family that is going through Tourette rages will be able to see themselves in that chapter and understand and know that we are people who have actually lived what they are living. The descriptions should make that very obvious. This is very intentional and meant to give them a sense that someone else in the world understands what it is like. The people around us, our friends, loved ones, and relatives struggled to grasp how hard it was for us. This left us feeling alone and desperate. A feeling I want to attempt to alleviate for others.

What you are about to read will hopefully resonate with you. It is our wish that at least one or two things will help you with this very complicated disorder. At no point do we want to convey that we are experts on every family and situation; however, we are definitely the most knowledgeable when it comes to our family and our experiences. We always recommend consulting with experts, doctors, and trained professionals as much as possible. But we also recognize the importance of learning from others who have gone through the same experience ahead of you.

It should be noted that our son Riley is also diagnosed with ADHD, OCD, anxiety, Executive Processing Disorder, Sensory Processing Disorder, and a myriad of other things. These comorbid diagnoses often occur with Tourette Syndrome. Many of the things discussed in this book can be applied to people struggling with just one or two of these diagnoses. The symptoms and behaviours are often very similar. The descriptions of what is happening in Riley's mind and body are straight from my son's mouth. It might shed some light on what is happening for your loved one too, even if they do not have Tourette Syndrome.

At the very least, we hope that Riley's lighthearted and intuitive personality draws you in and helps you learn and understand what's going on in his mind and body. Which will in turn give you the ability to better support and understand your child, student, coworker, classmate, or loved one with the diagnosis of Tourette Syndrome.

If you are reading this to a child and the child is upset by what happens with Riley, the best way to deal with this is through education and talking to them about their feelings. Help them to understand what life is like for Riley and how he must feel. I hope that this book will encourage our children, and adults, to be more understanding of this very difficult diagnosis. Especially when they encounter people with Tourette Syndrome in their schools, work places, and everyday life.

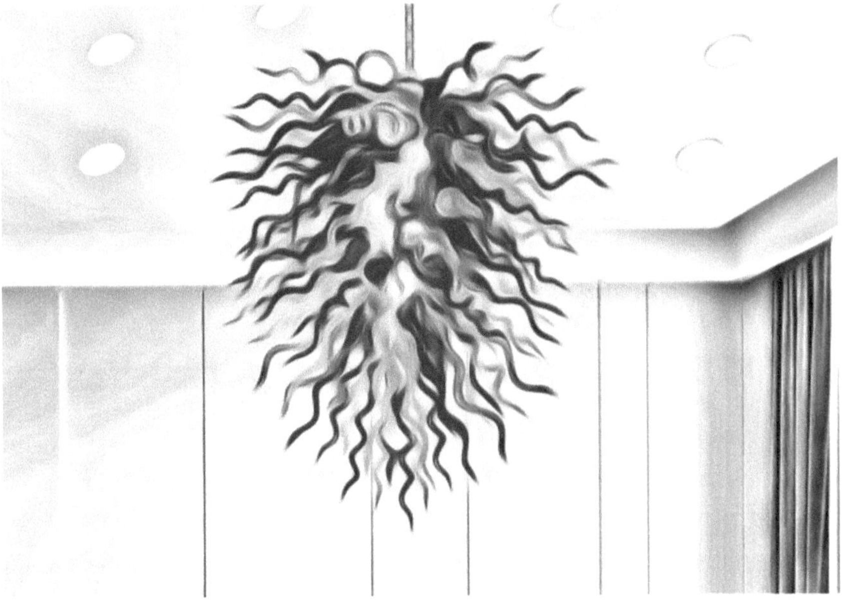

CHAPTER 1

THE BUMPY LUMPY LIGHT

Riley stood up in front of the class. He took a deep breath in and tried to focus on his story. He was a bit nervous, but he knew that all the other kids that had stood up in front of the class had likely been nervous too. He had enjoyed writing his story, and thinking of the fun he had with it gave him confidence in sharing it.

Riley took another deep breath and began. "In the middle of a square room, surrounded by square walls and corners, there is a bumpy, lumpy light. The light is a huge chandelier. A handblown glass display of beauty. It was made to bring an amazing coloured spectrum to the room. It is beautiful just as it was made. It has angles and branches coming off it. It has white and shades of blue colours in it. It is a masterpiece. It is one of a kind and completely unique.

"Surrounding this light are seven pot lights. They are white, round, and flat. They look and work just like each other. They are all the same. The same round white lights. They were created for a specific job too. They shine their bright light on the surfaces below them and make everything bright and easy to see. They function and act always as expected, all in unison.

"These round lights are together in a group. They have one another to identify with. They have things in common with each other. This makes them feel strong and good; better than the odd light in the middle of the room. The bumpy, lumpy light does not fit into their group. They think the chandelier is ugly and they don't mind telling it so on a regular basis. Mind you, they don't have a lot of other things to do. So, they occupy their time tormenting the bumpy light. They cannot believe it is in the centre of the room, on display almost! They say to the chandelier, 'Honestly, why would anyone put such a horribly shaped light in the middle of their room?' When they look at that light, they are slightly embarrassed! It is such a wild thing.

"They call the lumpy light names. They yell at the large light, asking it, 'Why are you so ugly and dumb?' But the chandelier was created differently than them and would reply, 'I am only different than you. Can you not see that? I was made to be in the centre of a room. I was made to be brilliant and shine everywhere; even up onto the ceiling. You are all made for a different purpose, and you don't work like me.' Often though, the chandelier felt lonely. It wished it had some other lights in its group. Lights that were like it. Lights that understood it and knew how it felt to be so unique. Sometimes the chandelier would wonder how it would ever be able to carry out its job of being such a special light. He would say to the round pot lights, 'You don't know what it's like to be me. I have lots of bulbs and take lots of energy to do what I do. I have to be kept shiny and clean to perform at my best. But my bumps, lumps, and branches are always getting dusty and dull. It is hard work making my light shine through all of that dust that collects on me. The people have to come and clean me all the time so that I shine my brightest. You need to understand that I have to be made different from you because my purpose is different.' The pot lights would just laugh at him and say, "Oh we don't want you around us. You don't fit into our group! You don't only look weird, but you make us feel weird. We don't like that.'

"The creator of the handblown glass light had made it very special. When it was first placed there, the room around it was still empty and bare. There were no other things in the room as it had just been built. Little by little, the room took shape around the light. Textures and fabrics were brought there to match the light—its colour, its brilliance, and its stature. The room came to life because of the chandelier. Furniture, paintings, curtains, carpets, and little itty bitty trinkets were all brought in to support the way the big chandelier made the room feel. That odd bumpy, lumpy light was made for this. It fulfilled its purpose by doing this.

"But the round pot lights continued to taunt the big light. They could not understand how such a strange looking light could be anything good. They asked, 'How could such a shape like that be good at being a light?' They really could not imagine that it had anything to offer anyone. They were the good lights. They belonged together, and after all, they were clearly the better choice. Why would anyone choose lots of them if they weren't the better choice? It was so glorious to be all alike. To fit in and adore each other. They did everything in unison together. That big ugly light was on its own circuit even. It turned off and on when they didn't! It couldn't even get that right! Such an obviously stupid light.

Finally the room was finished and the decorators were satisfied with the way it looked. The day of the room reveal came and a party was happening to celebrate. Someone came into the room and turned the pot lights on. They shone their brilliance down at the surfaces below. They performed all together and felt so proud. The people bustled around under their lights. They were dressed fancy and quickly went about arranging snacks, drinks, plates, bowls, and little itty bitty napkins. But something seemed not quite right. There were no comments made about the flat, white pot lights. No mention of how wonderful they did their job. Or how great it was that they were all alike. No one even noticed them, really.

The guests started to gather together and when everyone had arrived they were ready to show off the new room. Then the strangest thing happened; all the spotlights were turned off! But everyone was gathered around to see the new room! The pot lights couldn't imagine why they had been turned off. They thought, 'What on earth could be the point of that?'

"Then the unthinkable happened! The only light that was then turned on was the big chandelier hanging in the middle of the room. The people took quick breaths in. They oohed and aahed at the light. Some even stepped back a bit to get a better look. The beauty of the light could not be hidden. It was obvious to everyone there, even the pot lights. But try as they might to ignore it, this weird light was the centre of attention! This bumpy, lumpy light was suddenly the most important thing in the room. The pot lights heard comments like 'amazing,' 'incredible,' 'rare,' and the word they heard the most often: 'priceless.'

"The chandelier heard all the reactions to its light. It beamed with pride. It shone its light in the room to every corner and changed the look of the room. It radiated blue and white shades on every wall and the ceiling. It took people's breath away and made them all calculate in their heads how they could get one similar for their rooms. The handblown glass light knew it had finally become all that it had been created to be. Even though all the pot lights had shunned it since its arrival, it was the most perfect fixture to complete that room. The creator of that light, after all, had made it just for that room. With all of its weird angles, limbs, and colours, it was exactly what it was supposed to be. It was exactly what the pot lights were not!"

Riley stood at the front of the class. He felt good about the story and was happy he was able to share it. Ms. Ellsworth, his teacher, was looking at him with wide eyes.

She said to him, "Riley, where did you get that story?"

He replied, "I wrote it. But my mom helped me a bit with it. You know, all the right words and where to put the commas and such."

Ms. Ellsworth did not know what to say. She was shocked. She asked him where he got the idea for the story.

He replied, "One day I was standing in my kitchen, eating a snack. I was looking up at the ceiling for some weird reason and I noticed the pot lights in the ceiling. I saw how they all looked the same and worked the same way. Then I noticed some other lights hanging down on long posts. You have to use a different switch to turn those on. My mom said they were pendant lights. They were square and did not match the pot lights at all. I wondered about what it might be like if they could talk and whether or not the different lights would all get along and accept each other. So, I made it into a story. When I was done, I thought to myself that I am just like the bumpy, lumpy light. Most people around me are like the pot lights. And even though they do not think I belong, one day the things about me that make me unique will be the perfect fit. I know that right now they don't understand because they only see the surface of who I am. It's OK. I don't understand either some days."

Ms. Ellsworth was again speechless. Her mind was spinning with all that this little boy had stirred within her. She thought of all the children that she had taught before him that were just like Riley. Those children that she and everyone else had felt were odd or didn't fit in. How much of their potential had she completely missed because she had focused only on how they were different? She thought about how they made her feel frustrated because they couldn't learn the way she was trying to teach—the way she was taught to teach. In her insistence that every child fit a mold and be taught the same way, she was really excluding the children that were more unique and special than she could ever imagine. Their potential was completely missed because it seemed easier to try to make them fit into what was considered "normal." She wondered what it would take to help these kids be the best they can be and unleash their true potential.

"What first step can we take to make school work better for kids like Riley?" she wondered. Her heart felt heavy and sad, but she was determined to figure it out.

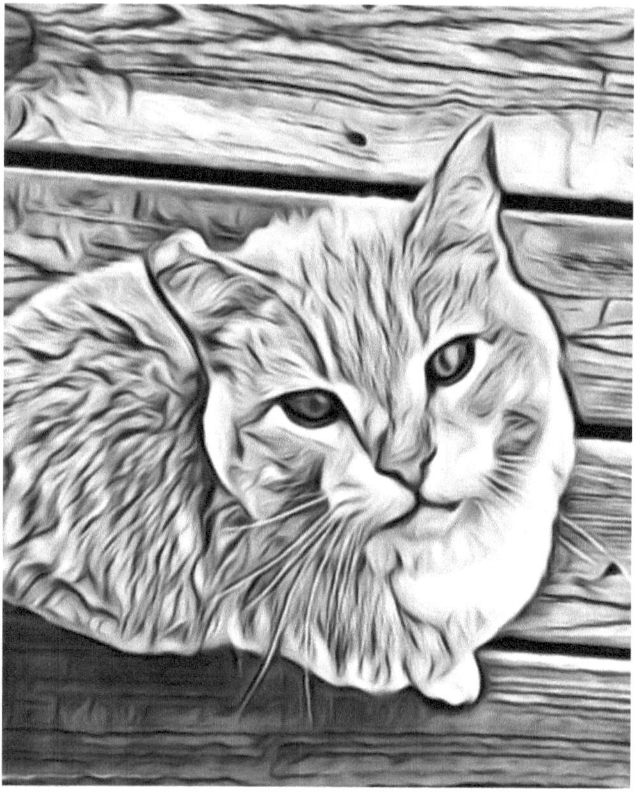

CHAPTER 2

CHARLIE

Riley ran all the way down the driveway when he got home later that day. He felt good about the story he had written. Everyone enjoyed his story. He most looked forward to telling Charlie, his cat, all about it. Charlie was a good listener. He was good at cuddles too. Riley liked that the most.

"My teacher was very surprised at my story," he relayed to Charlie. Charlie purred and kneaded Riley's leg with his paws. He was always happy to see Riley. "She doesn't seem to know that I don't fit in or why. I don't know why that is. But my family doesn't always understand me either, so it's OK." Riley laughed and snorted a bit. "Actually, I don't think I get it either." Riley lay down beside Charlie and sunk his fingertips into Charlie's soft fur. It felt so satisfying. Charlie smelled him with his wet nose and flicked the very tip of his tail.

Riley told Charlie all about the story. How he sometimes felt like a bumpy light amongst a bunch of round lights. That he often didn't feel like he fit into his classes and groups very well.

"You see," he told Charlie, "I have Tourette syndrome, and Mom says that Tourette syndrome often comes along with a whole bunch of other things too. It makes my body do tics. Those are repeating movements and sounds that are strange to people around me. She said I also have ADHD, OCD, executive processing disorder, and anxiety. I don't know what all those words mean, but I know that when they all come together, it makes me different from most of the other kids. It makes things go crazy in my brain too."

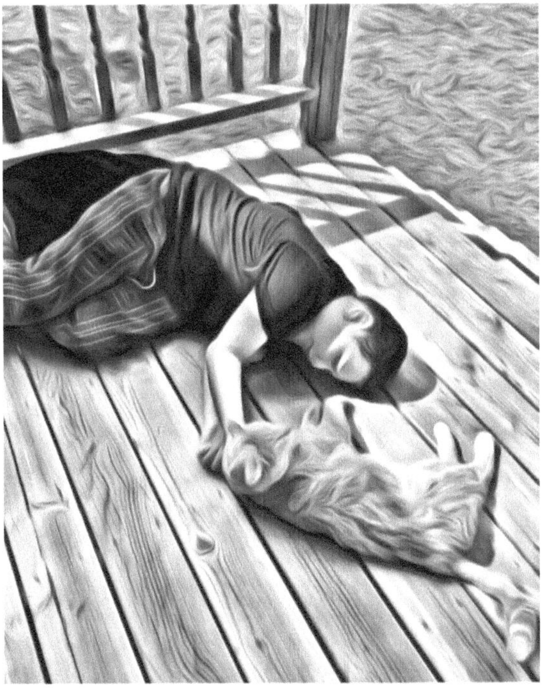

Riley began to tell Charlie all about Tourette syndrome. He figured Charlie probably knew all about it already, in his own cat way, but he made sure to tell him everything anyway. He told Charlie about his tics and how he can't really make them stop. Sometimes they make him do things that other people don't like. His tics make him make strange sounds and movements that the other kids bug him about.

"I don't know why I do those things, but I do," Riley explained to the listening cat. Riley sat for a minute and thought. Then Riley said his thoughts out loud. "You know, Charlie, it's weird, but when I am talking to you, my tics don't even happen. The same is true if I am watching TV or playing video games. Even when I am drawing. It sure is strange."

Charlie's tail tip swirled around and around as Riley talked. Sometimes he would flick it back and forth. Riley liked it when Charlie did that. It meant Charlie was happy. Riley lay back in the sun. Charlie curled up beside him. He liked the sun too. Riley continued his chat with Charlie. He told Charlie about how sometimes his brain asks him to do things and before he can even think about it, he is doing it. Or how sometimes he gets really worried about things and can't make his brain stop thinking about them. Like when his mom asks him to have a shower and it really upsets him. He loses control and gets really mad. She says it's because his brain is stuck on what he is doing and he has trouble switching gears. But Riley knows it's also because showering is hard. There are a lot of steps! It is a lot of work and it takes so long.

"The thought of it just makes crazy things happen in my mind and I don't like it," Riley explained to Charlie.

He didn't know whether other kids struggled like that or not, but he sure did. Sometimes his mom would ask him to clean up his room. He laughed and hugged Charlie tight.

He said, "Those are the hardest times of all. Cleaning my room. It's too much for me! Sometimes Mom doesn't understand why. It's just all the things everywhere. And my room is so big. It's a big list and so much work. Crazy things happen in my brain then too."

Riley picked at a mosquito bite. Charlie sniffed at what he was doing, flicked his tail, and lay back down beside him.

"Oh, that?" Riley asked Charlie. "Those are from the OCD, Mom says. It sure is a big urge for me. I can't stop picking at it for the most part. It just calls to me. I feel it there. I like the way it peels off under my nails. I find it very nice. Mom says I need to stop and it upsets her. But I don't think I can. We are trying to make it better. I need to try harder, Charlie. Maybe you can help me? You are a really good friend, Charlie. You always listen to me when I am upset. You are the best cat I could ever have.

"Mom thinks you are an angel in disguise sent to us. Dad thinks that you were sent to us on a mission. You sure came to us in a special way. That's for sure."

Riley gently touched Charlie's frostbitten ear. He had that when he came to their home. Charlie had wandered into their yard during the early spring of the Covid pandemic, and he had never left. It sure helped having a new friend when everyone was stuck at home. If the family was camping in the yard, Charlie would purr and meow at their tent. He wanted to come in with them. He would sit around the fire with them and keep everyone company. He loved being with the family. No one could figure out just how he had arrived there since he seemed to love his people so much. It seemed odd that he would have left his last home.

One time, Riley's dad said, "Maybe God was talking to Charlie and said that he had a special job for him. That he had a mission for Charlie to go on. I wonder if Charlie didn't want to go at first? Especially when God told him that he would have to wander through the countryside, be cold and hungry, and get a frostbitten ear?" Riley was sad when Dad said this part. Dad would continue and say something like, "Maybe Charlie told God he was willing to go if it meant he could help this little boy and his family. Charlie was willing to leave his family and his warm house to come help you, Riley, and to be with you."

Riley shook his head; he had tears in his eyes for Charlie's sake. He remembered the times when he was having a rage and the mere sight of Charlie would break him free of the rage. He would cry and cling to Charlie, and the fuzzy feline would never stop his hugs. Charlie would always sit still and let Riley hold him. This stray, orange-blonde cat that had wandered into their yard.

CHAPTER 3
MONDAY MORNING

It was a cool fall morning in the first month of school. Riley woke up to his mom gently shaking him.

"Riley. It's time to wake up for school," she said.

This morning it was hard to wake up. Riley had difficulty sleeping through the night. His weighted blanket had fallen off in the middle of the night, woke him up, and then he just couldn't get back to sleep for a long time. The other issue is that once he is awake, his tics start and those can be hard to stop. Sometimes his legs just won't stay still long enough for him to fall asleep. Then his brain starts obsessing over this or that and he is awake for hours.

Riley felt frustrated that he was so tired this morning and was being asked to wake up for school. He longed for a good night's sleep where he felt rested in the morning. Weekends were good for this as his mom would let him sleep as long as he wanted. Sunday nights were often the worst because he would be anxious about going to school the next day and about having to wake up early. As usual, last night was just that way. This Monday morning was turning out the same too.

But Riley forced himself to get out of bed. He was hopeful that it would be a great day in spite of how he felt. His arm tic started making his arm shoot out in front of him in a motion like a jet flying. He made a jet noise a few times, moved his arm again, and shook his head in rapid jerks that always went along with this tic. He ignored it all and went along with his mom to get some breakfast and get ready for school. His tics were really bad this morning, making him drop his toothbrush as his arm jerked out in front of him. It would be a long day of holding those tics in while he was at school. He felt tired and overwhelmed at the thought of it.

His mom interrupted his thoughts and asked him to focus and get ready for school. Riley was thankful for the quick pet he was able to give Charlie on his way to the bus. Charlie purred happily and enjoyed the scratches behind his ear. Whenever Riley scratched behind Charlie's ear, the cat's back leg would come up and start a scratching motion in the air right in time with Riley's fingers. "Oh, I've hit the good spot," he would say to Charlie. The interaction lifted Riley's spirits and he felt more hopeful about the day.

Riley was thankful that the morning was cool as it made the long bus ride easier to bear. He knew at the end of the day it would be hot and the ride would be long and difficult. He tried not to think about this and instead remembered how Charlie had purred loudly, so loud that his body was vibrating. Riley smiled and leaned his head against the window of the bus, closed his eyes, and tried his best to quiet his mind. His arm jerked out in front of him again and his head shook while his mouth made the jet sounds. After a minute of this, he settled back into his seat and drifted between being awake and asleep for a few minutes here and there, interrupted every now and then with another minute of his tics.

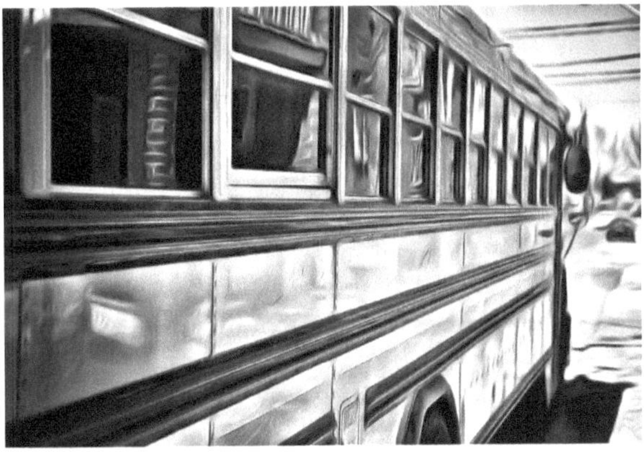

The noisy bus pulled up to the school. Riley was thankful that part of his day was over. The loud noises in the bus were very hard on his ears and his brain. They bothered him a lot, and he had forgotten to bring his earplugs. He didn't like using them anyway as the other kids could see them and that made him embarrassed. But the noises of the bus were so loud. Sometimes he would get mad at the kids and scream at them to be quiet. Most of the time he didn't bother as he knew it wouldn't help. They would all just get mad at him. He wondered why his bus had to be like this. Their old bus driver had never let kids be noisy on the bus. He missed her a lot. She was so good and so understanding. All the kids liked her so much and really behaved well on her bus. Now the bus rides were so long and difficult. Riley got off the bus and his head rapidly shook and twisted. His arm shot out.

Riley's first class was art. He was glad it wasn't math or gym. Those subjects were not his favourite. He struggled to learn math as it was hard to grasp all the steps and put them together. In math class, he always had to sit in his chair and not move around. This was hard because what the teacher was saying often didn't make sense to Riley and it made him anxious and fidgety. He would often get in trouble in math class.

Gym class only made him embarrassed as he just couldn't do all the things the other kids could do. When he tried, it usually went poorly. Sometimes his arm tic would make him drop the ball or throw it weirdly and the kids would laugh at him. Riley would trip over his own feet or not be able to handle a stick and a ball at the same time. Worst of all was that he had to change his shoes for gym class. He hated tying his laces and it was always a struggle for him. He wondered if he should ask Mom to get him different laces for these shoes, but he always forgot to ask her when he was at home.

But he loved art class. When he was drawing or doing art, his mind would be so focused and for a brief time, his tics would be gone. It was always a nice break from them, and he really enjoyed drawing. Riley felt good in art class as he was able to do things the way that made sense in his mind and worked well for him. The art teacher always encouraged them to follow her project, but to do it in a way that made it easy for them. She always showed them a couple of different ways to do things, and that helped Riley. He often couldn't do things the way the other kids did, but in art class it didn't matter, and no one noticed! He also didn't have to sit still in art and pay attention to the teacher at the front. She would only give one instruction and then let them catch up in their work to that point. Once he was caught up, Riley could wiggle in his seat or get up and move. It was easy in that class.

Suddenly, Riley's train of thought was interrupted by the intercom speaker in the room coming to life. It was loud and it scared him. It made his brain crazy with the interruption and how loud the sound was. His tics that he had been working so hard to control went crazy as his mind was overwhelmed by the noise of the speaker. The voice over the speaker bellowed out, "There will be a school assembly in the gym today after lunch. A short talk followed by a movie. Prepare to have fun!" Riley panicked inside. School assemblies were never fun for him. His arm jerked out in front of him again and again. His head shook and his mouth made the jet noise, over and over. He could not recover for the rest of art class. He was so frustrated and wanted to cry. He needed a break to calm down as he felt a rage coming in his mind. Riley asked his teacher to go to the break room, and he was allowed to go. His tics were all going crazy the whole way down the hallway. Even his eyes were rapidly blinking in sets of three blinks. He wanted to run to the break room, but knew he had to walk. In spite of all that was going on in his brain and body at this moment, as he walked he was careful to step on every third tile only. The break room was a safe place with padded floors, a swing, and a soft light. His brain needed a place to recover from what had just happened in art class … his favourite class.

Later that morning, Riley was making his way through math class. It wasn't easy, but as he looked at the clock, he was happy to see it was almost over. Ms. Ellsworth had been teaching something new and Riley really wanted to listen and pay attention, but he was struggling. His tics were overwhelming his brain, and his tired mind and body just wanted some kind of distraction. He couldn't understand what the teacher was saying or how to solve the question staring back at him from the page on his desk. Riley picked up his pencil and started his doodling. The tics and distractions would always get a bit better when he was doodling. He sketched around the questions on his math page, and it became a bit easier to listen to the teacher. That fidgety part of his brain was kept occupied by his pencil and the movement of his fingers as art came to life on his paper. Riley often got in trouble for doodling during class. His teachers didn't seem to understand that it kept part of his brain still and let the other part of his brain focus on his work. Today was no different.

Ms. Ellsworth called Riley's name and asked him to focus on the board and what she was teaching. Riley nodded his head as if he was going to comply. He kept doodling, hoping that she would just let him continue with what he was doing. She asked him to repeat to her what she had been talking about in an effort to see if he was indeed listening. He was able to repeat the last few minutes of the lesson, and this was strange to his teacher. But still, she was frustrated that he was drawing again and not watching the board.

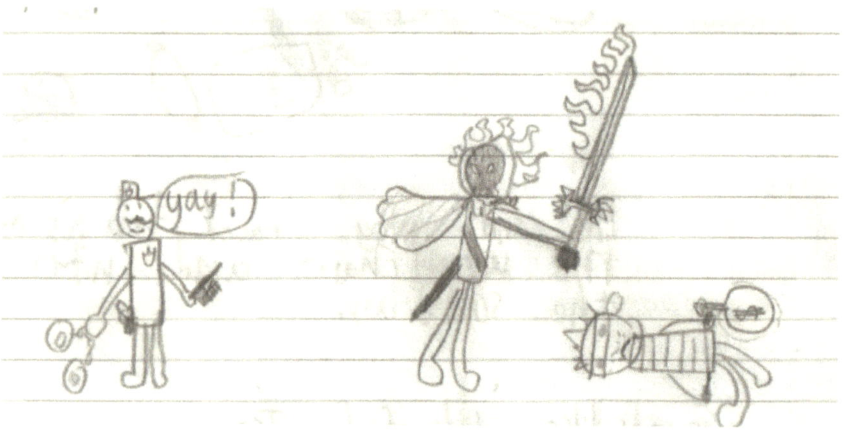

"Riley," Ms. Ellsworth called. "Please stop and pay attention or we will need to visit the principal's office for the rest of the class."

Riley stood up in frustration and said loudly, "I can't stop. I can't stop doodling!" He didn't know what else to say or how to explain it.

"Riley! Talking like that is something we cannot do, my friend. That is not OK." Ms. Ellsworth said. She asked Riley to head to the principal's office. He complied with her request to leave the classroom and was thankful to be walking down the hall, free of the demands of math class. He sure hated math class and felt sad Ms. Ellsworth was upset at him. But he didn't know what else to do. He wanted her to understand but couldn't figure out how to put it into words.

All through lunch hour, Riley was dreading the coming assembly. He was still so tired from last night and the day was getting long. He would never get control of his tics for the rest of the day now. He knew enough about his brain to know that it wasn't going to happen today. The kids eating their lunch around him were bugging him and telling him to stop making those noises and sounds. Even though they all knew that he had Tourette syndrome, they still were getting annoyed with him. They had all watched a video his mom had made for the class explaining his Tourette syndrome to them. Most of them had been in class with him since kindergarten. Honestly though, Riley was annoyed at his tics too! Very annoyed! So he tried his best to understand how it might be for the other kids to listen to his tics. He asked to go to the break room again. Hopefully it would help him get through lunch. At least no one would ask him to stop doing his tics in there.

When assembly time came, the gym was small. It had just enough room to fit all the students and staff without going over the fire safety regulation. The floor was hard and cold as there were no chairs set out for the kids. It was very noisy when Riley arrived to take a seat amongst the crowd. It hurt his ears. It made his head go numb and feel out of control. Their class sat down all together, and try as he might, Riley could not find a place on the edge of the row. He found himself sandwiched between other students. He was surrounded!

Riley began to obsess over how close everyone was. He felt closed in and wanted to run out of the gym. Everyone was being so loud and noisy, and he knew there was no room to do his tics. His brain was becoming very overwhelmed. The teacher at the front was talking about something, but he couldn't hear her. Part of his brain was trying to tell him to sit still and not do his tics, but another part of his brain was telling him to do his tics and was screaming so loud at him. The scream drowned out the teacher and overwhelmed him. He knew that scream well and had heard it often. He had even given it a name and called it "Eerie." Riley had explained to his mom one day that Eerie didn't stop screaming in his mind. It is always screaming at him to do his tics, except when he was reading or drawing, watching TV, or playing video games. That is the only time Eerie goes away for a bit. But right now, Eerie was louder than everything else in the room.

When the assembly movie started playing, Riley was able to be distracted enough that Eerie became less loud. He had gotten up and gone to the washroom and when he came back, he was able to sit at the very edge of the group, near the wall. This calmed his tics down a bit as he knew he could do them without disrupting anyone around him. Just because of this fact, he didn't feel the need to do them as much. But he still ticked through the whole movie. The kids around him glared at him for making noise and bothering them. Riley felt sad and frustrated, but he focused on the movie and looked forward to going home.

The bus ride home was loud again. Riley leaned his head against the window, trying to drown out the noise. He counted telephone poles as they drove by and the hour-long bus ride faded into the distance. The heat from the bus and kids squished in the seats exhausted him; he had to work hard to hold most of his tics in. But still his head shook, his arm shot out, his eyes blinked, and his mouth made the jet sound.

Walking down the driveway, Riley saw Charlie walking toward him. Charlie always greeted him when he came home. He petted Charlie, and the stress of his day started to melt away. His tics faded for a brief time, but he was still so exhausted. When Riley walked through the door, his mom greeted him and reminded him of the things he needed to do. He was so worn out from the day and didn't have the energy even to talk. His tics exploded now that he was home. Having held them in all day and having fought against Eerie all day, he suddenly gave in to the urge to do them and they took over his brain and body. His mom noticed how bad they were and wondered why. After he had put his lunch kit and shoes away, Riley asked his mom for video game time or TV time. He just wanted a break from his brain.

She replied, "Riley, I reminded you this morning that you need to have a shower today and clean up your room. Those things need to be done first."

Riley was powerless to stop what came next.

CHAPTER 4

ELISE

Elise Ellsworth, Riley's math and language arts teacher, lay her head on her pillow. "What a day this has been," she thought to herself. Her thoughts swirled. "Work sure was a challenge today. I really don't know about this feeling I have. This feeling that somehow I didn't get things quite right today with my choices and how things turned out." Her eyes closed as she drifted off to sleep. Her dreams were of battles and fights. She tossed and turned. It was a long night.

The next morning, Elise was getting a coffee in the staff room before classes began. She was tired from her restless night and her mind was wandering and somewhat off in dreamland still. Elise wrapped her hands around the warm coffee cup. The feeling was comforting and she leaned against the counter and sipped her coffee. She let her mind wander again as she contemplated what had upset her from the day before. While she was thinking, Sherri, the school's resident counsellor, came into the staff room. Sherri looked at Elise and could tell by the look on her face that Elise was deep in thought. In fact, she had not even noticed that someone had entered the room.

She said to Elise, "Wow, you seem pretty far away. Is everything OK?"

Elise chuckled and replied, "Oh yes, I'm fine. I didn't have a good sleep last night because I was thinking about a situation in my math class yesterday with one of my students, Riley. I'm going over it in my mind, trying to get it figured out."

Sherri said, "Why don't we meet for lunch later? Maybe we can talk about it and figure it out together." Elise liked that idea and the two agreed to meet for lunch.

When Sherri and Elise met for lunch, they began talking about what had troubled Elise from the previous day. The difficult math class with Riley flashed into her mind and her stomach made that flutter when you know you have hit on the very thing that is making you feel upset.

She said to Sherri, "It's hard as a teacher because the kids look up to you so much to always get things right. It's a huge pressure. Most of the time I think we do get things pretty good but then there are times when we know we totally dropped the ball. I think the way I handled Riley yesterday was one of those times." Sherri nodded as she devoted her attention to Elise.

Elise continued, "I am trying to wrap my head around just what it is that I need to understand with Riley. There is a huge block in my mind when I try to process just what it is I need to do to help him be successful ... especially in math class. He really struggles with not only the subject but the class itself. In language arts he seems to do much better. I've talked to his other teachers and they said he does have some difficulties here and there, but nothing like I see in math class. His art teacher has the most positive feedback about how he manages in her class."

Both Elise and Sherri sat quiet for a few minutes as thoughts and feelings swirled in their minds. Both were contemplating all that they knew and had experienced through their years working with students and the difficulty facing them with Riley.

Sherri broke the silence first and said, "I have talked with Riley many times. He is such a positive kid but he definitely has a lot going on behind those eyes. Super complex disorders that must give him a lot of challenges throughout his days. My guess is that each class and topic offers different hurdles for him to overcome. He does have a diagnosed math learning disorder; combined with the ADHD and Executive Processing Disorder affecting his ability to sit still, concentrate, and not get overwhelmed by all the steps in math, I think it takes over his brain sometimes. I wonder if we should be amazed that he can absorb anything we are teaching him when so many other things are going on in his mind at the same time?"

Both ladies pondered this thought for a few minutes. Sherri spoke again and said, "I'm getting this idea in my mind. The thing that makes it most difficult for us to help kids like Riley is the fact that all of his disabilities are going on behind the scenes. There is no flashing light or sign on his head telling us when he is struggling or having a difficult day. We are only left to guess as to why he is acting a certain way or doing a distracting thing like doodling. There is really no outward sign that we are asking him to do something he truly cannot. The only way we know that he isn't having success at what he has been asked to do is after the fact; when he wasn't able to do it and substituted it with something like doodling on his page. In reality, it often isn't until days later when we mark his paper that was handed in."

Elise eagerly nodded her head in agreement. She looked down at the table as she thought about what Sherri had said. Her mind was swirling with all kinds of thoughts. She felt a bit overwhelmed at trying to put it all together. She was thankful for the chat with Sherri; between the two of them, they just might be able to figure this out.

Sherri continued. "Picture this," she said to Elise, "Imagine if there was a student that was in a wheelchair because his legs were paralyzed. Imagine if he went to gym class and the teacher was asking the students to run laps up and down the bleacher stairs to warm up. The student in the wheelchair wasn't given any other options, so sitting at the bottom of the stairs looking up at them was the only thing he could do. The gym teacher walks over to him and asks why he is just sitting there and tells him to get busy doing his laps. So the confused student starts wheeling his chair around the gym, because what else could he do? Then the teacher comes over to him again and sends him to the office because he wasn't doing as instructed. The class was going to be playing floor hockey and needed to really warm up their legs and the student in the chair was only warming up his arms by wheeling his chair around. The teacher sends him to the office because he is not following instructions and causing a disruption in class. That scenario sounds super weird, right? What teacher would do such a thing?"

Elise nodded her head in agreement and wondered where on earth Sherri was going with this. But something about what Sherri was saying began to come together in her mind. She put her hand under her chin and listened intently for what Sherri would say next.

Sherri added, "Essentially we are doing the same thing to kids like Riley. In all honesty, it is just as weird if you think about it. It is not because we are trying to be insensitive, but like any student with learning disabilities or mental processing disabilities, it is super hard to figure out sometimes. We teach them the same way, ask them to read the same text books, ask them to take the same tests and sit in the same classes in the same structure as all the other students. When they are unable to do that, they come into conflict with our system in all different kinds of ways. Whether it be low marks or trips to the principal's office; we punish them on a regular basis for not being able to do what everyone else can do. But as I mentioned before, it is very difficult to assess in the moment what is going on for them; it's not like an orange light flashes when they can't do a math problem and a blue light flashes when they are starting to have trouble focusing. A teacher would never normally ask a child in a wheelchair to climb a set of stairs, but at the same time, asking Riley to overcome all of the obstacles that happen for him in math class is basically the same thing; we just can't visually see it."

Sherri paused for a bit and then said, "You know, our education system is built to teach all kids in the same way and has been that way for centuries. But in the middle of a class or a lesson, it is hard to remember that something a child might be doing cannot be seen in the same way as another child doing the identical thing. With thirty kids in our classes, it can be hard to keep all that floating in our mind. In a split second reaction in response to a behaviour, we can easily default to how we respond to every student that might be doing the same thing. However, this is definitely something we need to get out of the habit of doing and train ourselves to look for other indicators and outward signs that tell us what is going on behind the scenes at that moment."

Elise rubbed her face and forehead with her hands. She felt the heaviness of this as she knew it applied to more kids than just Riley. But she had trained for this. Part of her education taught her about this and taught her how to problem solve. It still felt pretty huge, and while she felt like it might just be something she would never be able to manage, she remembered her training and how in the past she had succeeded at solving puzzles like this by starting with one step, one piece. She wished her university education had far more info on Tourette syndrome than it did. "I think it wasn't even more than a paragraph!" she thought to herself.

She sat up straight and thanked Sherri so much for chatting with her and listening to her. She announced to Sherri, "The first thing I'm going to do is call Riley's mother. If anyone knows some signs to watch for when Riley is struggling, it's her. I'm also going to ask his other teachers to remember a time when he struggled in their class and what it looked like. If they can't remember a time, then I will ask them to watch for one and jot the details down for me. I can also have a chat with Riley. Maybe he and I can come up with some ways of making math class a bit more manageable for him. Maybe he can help me understand what it looks like on the outside when he is getting overwhelmed or what it is that he does to cope. But most of all, I honestly need to apologize to him for how I handled yesterday. Explain to him that teachers make mistakes too, but that I want a fresh start. Hopefully going forward, him and I can work as a team instead of against each other."

The ladies went their separate ways but thanked each other for the great chat.

Elise was walking into her classroom when she ran into Riley. "Good afternoon, Riley," she said. Riley gave a hearty "good afternoon" back to her. Yesterday's struggle with this incredible student and his doodling in class came flooding back to her. She thought about Riley and what she had read in his file. Tourette spectrum disorder. For Riley, this included symptoms associated with ADHD, OCD, anxiety, executive processing disorder, and Tourette syndrome. She knew he also had issues with social skills, learning math, and gross and small motor coordination. The difficulty with a diagnosis like Riley's is that it is all going on behind his sweet little face. Her mind was spinning about how little she knew about what life was like for Riley. How little she knew about how to help him. How do they reach out to a little guy like him? How do they stop asking him to do everything the other kids do without making him feel like he doesn't belong? It was so easy to treat Riley the same and have the same expectations of him when his disabilities were invisible and he looked just like every other kid on the outside. Her mind wrestled with the idea that they were demanding that he achieve the same standards and grades as kids that did not have any medical or learning diagnoses. Her mind remembered the example Sherri gave about the student in the wheelchair. But at the same time, they wanted

Riley to strive to learn, and encourage him to want to achieve what the other kids were doing. They wanted to help him learn from being around his friends and groups of lots of other students with all kinds of different personalities. Where was the happy middle ground in this?

When she had a spare moment, Elise emailed her principal to make an appointment with her. She would need help in piecing this all together.

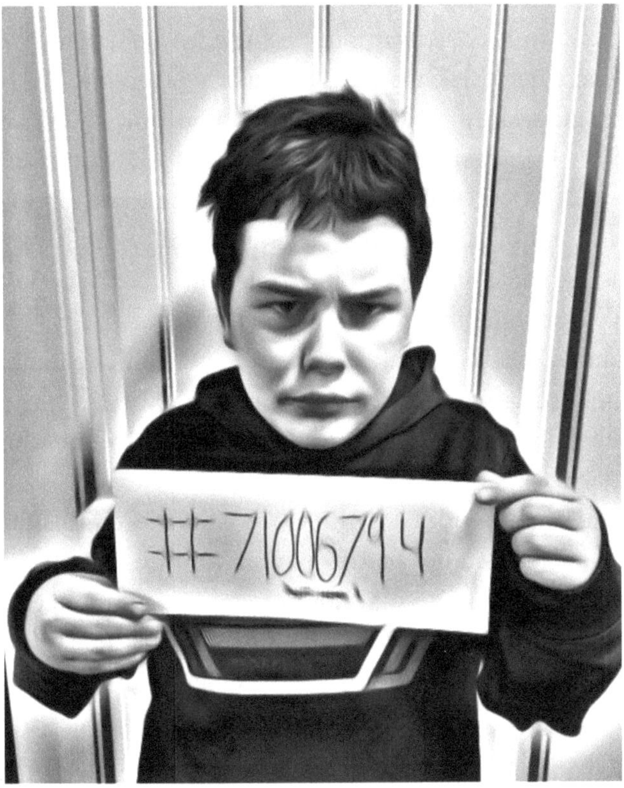

CHAPTER 5
WHAT CAME NEXT

Riley could feel his mind spinning out of control. He knew this feeling well. It happened lots. It was Tourette Rage attacking him again. His mom's request that he shower and clean his room was more than his brain could handle at that moment. His OCD kicked in, and over and over the voice in his mind told him that he just wanted video games! The necessary mental and emotional transition that he had to make from the bus and school to being at home was beyond his reach now, never mind a shower!

Riley could no longer hear his mom as the familiar rage engulfed his mind. He tried to keep it away, but he knew it would win. It was always scary for him when this happened. He quickly faded into the back of his mind. He could hear himself scream at his mom and say he hated her! It made him cry inside, but he was unable to stop it. His stomach churned with anxiety as he knew where this was going. The adrenalin was flooding his body and mind, making him lose even more control over his words and actions. He could no longer think straight or affect his actions at all; he was a helpless prisoner in his own mind and body.

His mom reacted to the things he was saying. She demanded to know what was going on. Why was he acting this way?

She said, "Riley! You need to stop talking to me this way; it is unacceptable!"

His mother had no idea why they had entered into this place at this moment. She had tried her best to remind him this morning, and even yesterday, that he would need a shower today. It was Tuesday, and cleaning his room and showering were what they did on Tuesdays. Having the schedule helped Riley know what was coming. She had set this up with him to help him be able to transition to getting things done. But even still, this rage was coming from out of the blue. Her anxiety increased as Riley screamed at her. They had been through this so many times before. Her adrenalin was hitting her mind and body too as the familiar movie played itself out in her home. She felt so exhausted. "Where is this coming from?" she wondered again.

Riley threw a book at her and threw down a shelf. His mom tried to stay calm and asked him to go to his room and find some calming things to do. She was getting nervous over the things he was doing. She needed some space between them. But Riley would not stop. He would not leave. Inside, Riley was so scared. He wanted his mom more than anything right now. He needed her hug, her soft words, but she would not give them to him. She could not give them to him as her anger and hurt overwhelmed her. He was crying inside and shaking. He only wanted her near him and to be close to her. Instead, he watched in horror as he screamed at his mother and told her he wanted her to die! Riley was a captive in his own brain. An observer in a prison cell, watching things go down outside his cell door. His brain had lost control over what he was doing and the storm inside his mind raged on.

Riley's mom said to him in a loud and angry tone, "Riley, you are not getting video games tonight, and if you don't stop, you won't get video games tomorrow either! Get into your room and do the things you need to do so that you can calm down!"

Riley's brain spun deeper into the storm. He screamed at her in reply, "I hate you! I'm going to punch you!" He threw down more items and threw another book at her.

She marched over to him and commanded, "That is enough! You need to go to your room! This type of behaviour is not OK! When you feel like this, and are acting like this, you need to take yourself to your bedroom and stay there until you can act appropriately!"

She dodged a toy that was a missile aimed at her. She grabbed Riley and half picked him up and half walked him to his room.

Once in his room, Riley could hear his mom crying on the other side of the door. He wished so much that this would stop. But in dismay he watched himself kick his door and scream at her. He was getting tired, but the storm in his mind was still raging. He could faintly hear his mom remind him to grab a book to read or some paper to draw with. Riley wanted to do these things, but he was still locked behind the bars of his mind.

His mom said, "Riley, you need to stop! Why don't you find a stuffy to cuddle or do the breathing exercises?" There was now a small crack in the door and Riley replied to her requests with another kick aimed right at that crack.

A short pause in activity gave Riley's mom a chance to leave the door. She had also given up that this would end right now with how she was handling things. She knew what she was doing wasn't helping, but her brain had been overwhelmed with emotions and adrenalin. She was no longer able to think straight. It had already been over two hours since Riley's rage had started. She was so exhausted, but still a thought came to her. A small glimmer of hope.

Riley's mom went quickly outside and called, "Charlie, Charlie!" Even though she was allergic to the cat, she knew it would help Riley snap out of the place he was in. Charlie came around the corner of the house, meowing. He was happy to see her and even though they rarely saw him run, he broke into a cat trot and meowed again. Riley's mom picked him up and kept him at arm's length, even though that is not how cats like to be carried. But Charlie didn't struggle or try to get away. He just hung there as she carried him into the house. He wasn't normally allowed in the house due to her severe allergies, but she didn't care at that moment. Riley meant more to her than her dumb allergies and the rash she would have later.

She called out to Riley, who was quieter now. "Riley, there is someone here to see you!"

Riley yelled, "Go away and leave me alone! Shut up!"

She put Charlie down and opened the door quietly. Then she picked Charlie up and put his head around the door to peek in at Riley. Riley saw Charlie and started to cry. Charlie meowed loudly. Riley reached for the big cat and took him in his lap. Riley cried and cried as he petted the purring feline. Charlie sat quietly in Riley's lap and let him hug him and stroke his fur. Charlie looked around at his sudden placement in the house and meowed at Riley, purred, and kneaded his paws on Riley's legs.

Outside, Riley's mom shook with relief as she hoped this would end the rage for today. Some of the things she had learned in the past were able to make their way through the fog in her brain. Under a bit more control now, she remembered that she needed to not talk to Riley right now and give him some space to just focus on Charlie. She left the two alone and went to her room to calm down. She sat on her bed and cried. So many thoughts and feelings flooded her mind and soul. The adrenalin leaving her body made her feel weak and tired. Knowing she hadn't handled the whole thing well, she cried even harder and longed for better days. She loved her boy so much. She hated these times and the damage they did to their home, their son, to her, and to their relationship. She hated Tourette syndrome and all the things that went with it. She hated what it did to her boy! She was grateful that Riley's younger sister was visiting a friend today so that she didn't have to go through watching another rage happen.

Riley's dad arrived home from work. He was pretty surprised to see Charlie in the house. But when he looked around and saw the things thrown about the house, he knew what had gone on. He felt sad inside and overwhelmed. Peeking in on Riley, he saw Riley and Charlie were OK. He went to find Riley's mom and saw she was recovering, and he hugged her. Going back to Riley in his room, he bent down to talk to Riley.

"How are you doing, kiddo?" he asked. "How did Charlie open the door and get in here with you?" Riley's dad knew that well timed humour and joking almost always helped Riley come out of his rage. Sometimes they would even turn a comedian on or a favourite funny TV show so that Riley would laugh and be able to break out of his rage. Riley smiled a tiny smile at his dad and hugged Charlie more.

He said, "Dad, you better take Charlie out so that mom doesn't get sick." Dad helped Charlie out of the house and gave him a nice scratch behind his ear. The rage was over for now. It was time to fix what had been done.

CHAPTER 6
CLEANING UP

Riley's dad went back to Riley's room after checking on Mom again. He stopped short when he reached for the door handle. Frustration and anger flooded his heart when he saw the growing hole in Riley's door that he had not noticed earlier. He felt himself crumbling under the weight of all that was going on. The long hours he put in at work were just enough for them to get by, and now he had to replace this door too! He wanted to scream and yell at Riley! Scream and yell at what their lives had become. He felt so hopeless and overwhelmed. He tried his best to push those thoughts aside and took a few minutes to calm down. He needed to get back to the place where he could talk to Riley. Riley's dad took a few deep, slow breaths.

"What happened today, Riley?" his dad asked him. Riley replied by telling his dad about his day. He became upset again when he was talking about the assembly and the bus rides. He told his dad about his not-so-great sleep the night before and that he knew it would be a hard day in the morning because he was so tired. Plus, he said, his tics were already out of control in the morning, and he could tell by the schedule they were on that they would be bad all day. Riley's dad hugged him and said he was sorry that he had such a rough day.

They continued to talk. Riley's dad said, "You know, Riley, we know you pretty well and I imagine your teachers are getting to know you pretty well too. But even though that's true, we still cannot read what is going on in your brain and we don't know what the day has been like for you. It is really important that you share that stuff with us. Even when it is difficult to do so. You could always write it in a note or even draw it in a cartoon for us. We can't read your mind and we need your help to understand what is going on for you."

Riley nodded. He knew all that, but today he had not been able to voice how he felt. "I'm sorry, Dad," Riley said. "I was just in a fog all day and didn't do a good job of telling anyone about that. I hurt Mom. How can I fix that?" Riley cried and his dad hugged him.

"It's OK, Riley," Dad said. "Mom still loves you and I know that you love her. Yes, your words and actions did hurt her, but I am pretty sure she will forgive you. I bet there are things that she might like to say sorry for as well. Did you want to go chat with her too?"

Riley nodded his head and got up to go talk to his mom. He was dreading it but knew it had to happen.

He found his mom reading a book to his little sister who had just arrived home. He asked if he could talk with her. His mom was dreading this part too, but also knew that they needed to try their best to fix things.

"Mom, I am sorry for the way the day went today," Riley said. "It was a bad day right from the start. I'm sorry for the things I said and did. Please forgive me."

Mom smiled and pulled him close. "I know, Riley," she said. "I forgive you. Can you forgive me for screaming and not understanding or trying to figure out what else might be happening? I didn't do a good job of supporting you. I'm sorry for that. Plus, some of the things I learned in the past just left my brain when you started screaming at me and throwing things at me. I didn't make good choices the whole time either. Maybe we can both try to do better the next time?"

Riley nodded. Tears rolled down both of their cheeks. Riley wiped his tears and hugged his parents. He then had to go and pick up the things he had thrown around the room. He hated this part; it made him frustrated. But he knew his parents would not let him skip this. After all, it was him that made this big mess no matter the reason it happened. As he picked up the books he had thrown, he wondered just how to make these rages go away.

While the leftover bad feelings from the rage were not fully gone, Riley was able to smile again and finished the night on a positive note. Dad joked again about how Charlie must have figured out how to open the front door and get in the house. The kids laughed at the thought of this.

"Well, after all," Dad said, "Charlie does have what looks like a thumb on his front paws. Maybe this gives him special powers?"

Mom and Dad helped Riley tidy up his room just so that he could go to sleep. Riley would need to tackle the rest of it the next day. His mom suddenly remembered that Riley still had not showered either. She sighed and thought to herself, "No one will die if he doesn't shower today. We will try again tomorrow. Hopefully he has a good sleep tonight and then tomorrow he will be able to manage that."

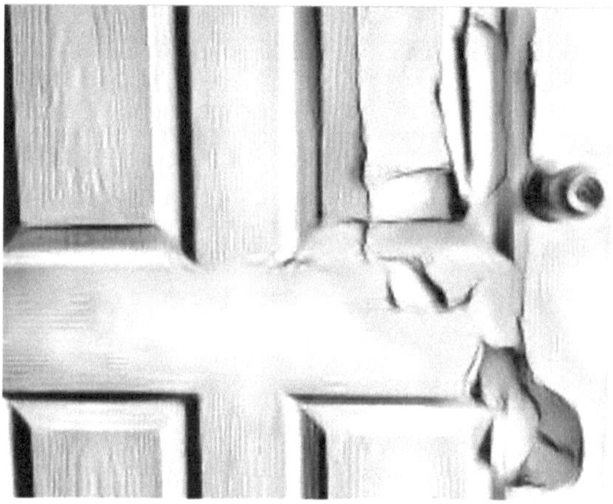

The next morning, everyone started the day on a fresh note. Riley's parents had sat together for their morning coffee. They prayed together and asked God to give them wisdom and the ability to manage this season of their lives. They talked about how the day had gone yesterday and his mom cried over the things she felt she had messed up when handling the situation. But still, forgiveness had given them all the courage to face another day. They still felt frustrated, a bit hopeless, and overwhelmed. However, they pushed those thoughts and feelings to the side and did their best to focus on the positives and start with a new day.

Riley had a good sleep that night due to the exhaustion from the day before and the rage. He felt better today. He looked at his broken door and his messy room and felt sad. But he knew that he could clean it when he got home. His brain was settled this morning, and his tics were still there but not as frequent. His arm shot out and his head shook as he thought, "Yep, still ticking, but on a good schedule today. I should be able to handle them at school." Everything was going better that morning and Riley gave Charlie a pet as he walked to the bus. He remembered how the cat had

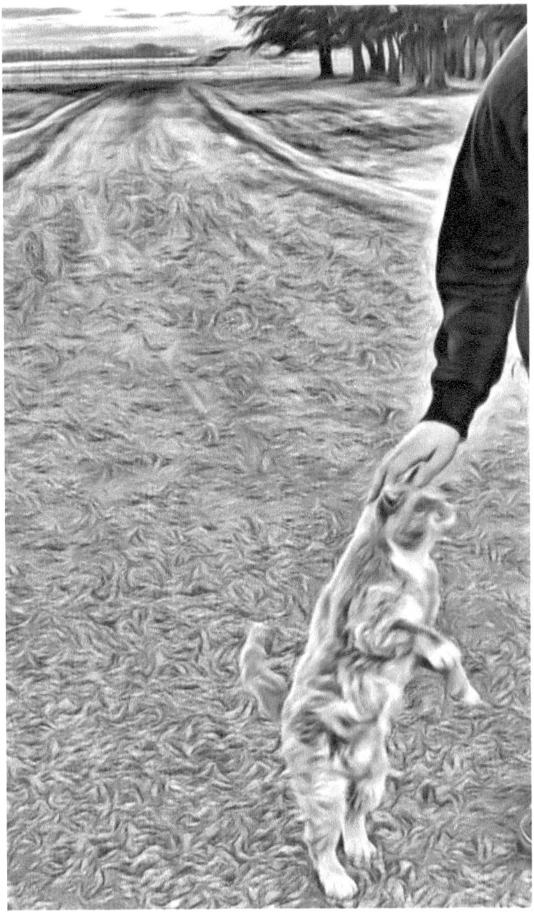

saved him yesterday. He loved Charlie so much. Charlie and his frostbitten ear. The cat stood up on his hind legs to receive the pet from Riley and meowed loudly. Charlie always walked to the bus with them and today he trotted happily alongside Riley.

Riley silently wondered to himself, “Does Charlie know what happened yesterday? Does he remember suddenly being in the house and in my lap?” Riley laughed to himself. “I bet that was quite a shock for him! Charlie is probably trying to figure out how he can get that to happen again and on a more permanent basis.”

At school, Ms. Ellsworth greeted Riley. He seemed a bit brighter today. She noted Riley was having a much better morning. Riley told her how his dad had made a joke about Charlie opening the door and coming into their house on his own. That Charlie was an outside cat but he had been allowed inside for a bit last night, and did she know that Charlie has a thumb on his front paws? Ms. Ellsworth wasn’t sure how all that happened, or about the thumb on his front paws, but Riley seemed focused on the quirky events with his cat. Riley’s arm shot out and he made his jet sound. The class was unaffected by this. For the most part, they had all gotten used to these noises and sounds from Riley. His head jerked and his eyes quickly blinked three times, but he managed to pay attention in spite of them.

Ms. Ellsworth had no idea what had happened at Riley's house the night before, or even what had brought the change in Riley from yesterday to today. Some days he seemed like such a different kid. The tics were always there, but some days he could sit still and pay attention and other days he just seemed to be somewhere else, unable to focus on any task. She thought to herself that she really needed more information on the struggles he has. Maybe today would be a good day to call his mother and see what went on over the last forty-eight hours. Yesterday was hard for Riley for some reason. "I sure would like to be able to make things easier for us and him," she thought. "I need to look up Tourette syndrome and see what it is about it that makes this more than just tics. It sure seems like there is more going on here than just tics." These thoughts went on in her head while she got the class started on their math for the day.

Later that day, Ms. Ellsworth talked with Riley's mom. They each shared what the last couple of days had been like for both of them. They expressed their frustrations and thoughts on how things had played out. Riley's mother talked about how a lot of what happened really came out of the blue for her. But as she listened to the events that had happened at school that day, the rage that Riley had when he arrived home began to make more sense. Riley's mother explained to his teacher about how the events at school would have felt for Riley. She was able to tell Elise about the fact that Riley struggles with sleep and how when he is tired, everything is much more difficult for him; he just isn't mentally refreshed enough to keep everything in balance. She discussed with Elise how Riley's anxiety and OCD come crashing together when he is put in a situation like an assembly, and how they might be able to manage it better for him in the future.

Added to the mix is Riley's need to do his complex motor tic with his arms, which would be difficult to do when he is squished into a gymnasium and given very little space. Not being able to do these tics would only make things worse and the struggles in his mind would pile up from there. She talked about how exhausted Riley can get from trying to keep everything in balance in his mind. "He really wants to make a good impression on his teachers and his classmates," his mother explained. "He holds everything together as best he can all day at school, and many days he barely makes it. When one extra thing like an assembly is added, he simply gets buried under it all. But often, unknown to most of us around him, many things are added to his day that make things more difficult for him."

Riley's mom started to share a thought with Elise that had occurred to her many times before. She said, "You know, the thing that makes this the most difficult for kids with intellectual and emotional disabilities is that it is all going on behind the scenes. For the most part, Riley seems to be doing fine on the outside, and those around him have no idea that he is struggling until he lets it explode. We have explained to him many times that he needs to share what's going on in his mind and heart when he is getting overwhelmed with things, and then also try to get to the root of why it is that he is having difficulties. We have talked with him about how important it is for him to be open with people so that they can support him, and how we can't read his mind."

Elise agreed, and she talked about how hard it can be to figure out that Riley is overwhelmed.

Riley's mom added, "It would be much easier if a child had a broken leg or was in a wheelchair. If you see that physically challenged child sitting at the base of a staircase, or something like that, looking at the staircase and trying to figure out how they will get up the stairs, you as an outsider would immediately be able to tell they needed help with that. It would also be super weird if you somehow expected that child to 'get over it' and get mad at them for not getting up the stairs or expect them to just figure it out. They would need assistance or a change in the situation somehow and simply are not able to physically do it. But for people like Riley, those outward signs of struggle are just not there, and those of us around them are left to guess and attempt to figure it out."

Elise had shivers going up her spine and goosebumps on her arms as Riley's mother talked about the staircase. Her conversation with Sherri at school flashed back into her mind. She told Riley's mother about what Sherri had said and they were both shocked at how similar it was to what Riley's mother had just said. The two shared thoughts on how much they wanted to make changes that would help these children be more successful with the minds they were given. "But what is the key?" they both asked.

They talked about the doodling in class. Riley's mother was able to piece the doodling together with Elise. Riley had often talked about the need to doodle and how it helps him focus. Riley's mother laughed as she said, "Sometimes I find Riley sitting at the table listening to music, drawing, and watching a video on drawing all at the same time! It is almost like the busy part of his brain requires that extra thing going on in order for him to sit and listen to what you are saying. We have talked with him about fidget toys and other items that he might utilize during class to keep that restless part of his brain busy."

Elise added a "yes" in agreement.

Riley's mom continued. "However, I think if you watch closely, you will notice that the doodling occurs most when Riley has come up against a question or problem in math that he doesn't know how to do. The minute he cannot continue his work, he starts doodling. It looks to the teacher like he is still working; however, he has simply given up on answering the question and is now just entertaining himself. There is definitely a difference in the purpose of doodling there." Riley's mother shared how they had explained to Riley that when he is doodling, he needs to keep his drawings simple and easy. That if he allows the drawings to become complex and detailed, it will no longer be a helpful tool and will then become a distraction. They had asked Riley to pay close attention to that and make sure that he kept the drawings light and easy.

Elise expressed appreciation for all the extra information and said that she would be sharing these beneficial tips with the rest of the staff that interact with Riley. The two agreed to have a meeting later in the week to share more thoughts and ideas of how they could make things better going forward. With a heavy heart, Elise added the need to apologize to Riley for not really getting it.

Riley's mother replied, "Don't be too hard on yourself. He will understand. He has to put up with it from his parents all the time! We so often just do not know, or we don't handle things right. But I appreciate so much that you are trying to make things better for him. I hope we can come up with some great ideas and plans to make things easier for everyone."

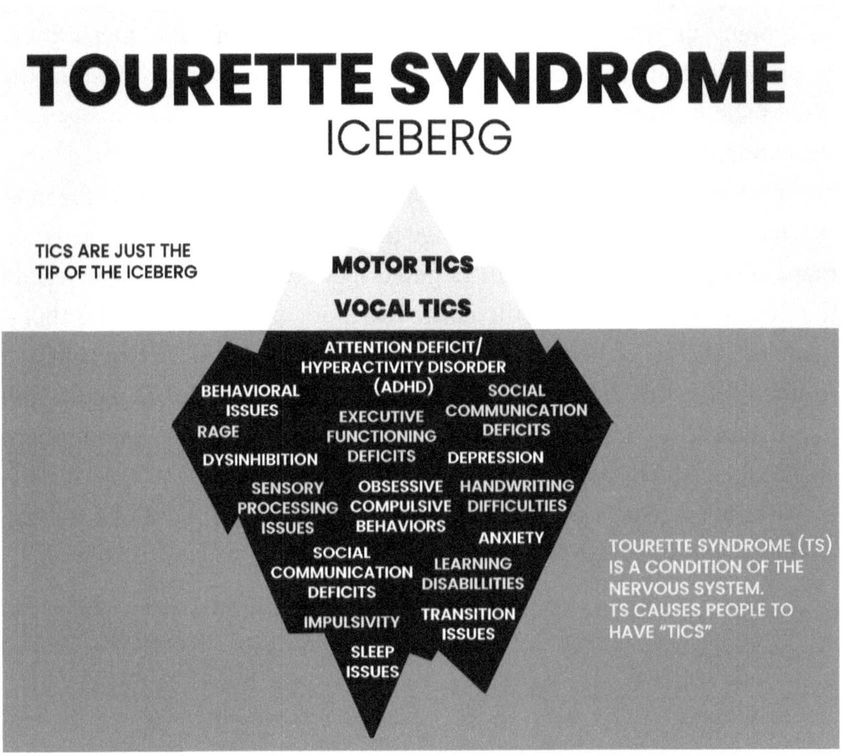

Later that day, Elise Ellsworth looked up Tourette syndrome, and a picture came up of an iceberg. She learned about how people with Tourette syndrome struggle with a lot more than just tics. She knew from Riley's file that there were a lot of things the doctor had diagnosed him with. She read more about the disorder, and in doing so, realized how much Riley must struggle with in his mind. A thought occurred to Elise. Her mind worked hard to grasp it all. She thought to herself, "Riley is actually a pretty good student. His marks aren't horrible, and he comprehends most of what I tell him. He does not do too bad on his tests, and because of that he must hear and retain most of what I tell him." She let that sink in for a few minutes. "Wow!" she thought. "He really has an amazing brain. With all the things he has going on inside that mind of his in a day, he still learns and retains the information we give in class. Honestly, that is a bit mind-boggling. How does he even do that? That brain is not a disabled brain, it is an amazing brain! What a strong kid!"

Elise's perspective on Riley was slowly changing. Even though there were many difficult days with Riley, she was suddenly able to see them in a new light. It gave her a lift in her spirit, and she thanked God for the insight she had just been given. She hoped it would help her change how she handled Riley and worked with him. She would share these things with his other teachers and their principal. Maybe they could work together as a team to figure out how to change their expectations of what he could manage or do. To see his brain as gifted in so many ways. To manage all the things that he did and still learn. The thought of it was so wild that it made her shake her head and smile to herself and think, "I have so much to learn!" But she felt hopeful that things would start to get better and that maybe this could be the beginning of something great! That thought excited her. Overwhelmed her really. Because she knew that if she was embarking on what God had planned, the possibilities would be beyond anything she could ever imagine!

CHAPTER 7
CARRYING ON

That night, Riley was able to have his shower. His day had been much lighter and although the noisy, hot bus still was a bit too much, he was able to ignore it by putting his headphones on and listening to music. Riley was smiling and laughing when he came in the door, and his mother knew this was a good sign.

"Charlie met us on the driveway!" Riley and his sister exclaimed. "Then he rolled around in the gravel and just lay there in the middle of the driveway! He is such a cat. Just lies down wherever and it doesn't matter that it is right in the middle of the road! Then he just looks around at us as if to say 'what? Pet me already!'" Riley shook his head at the silly cat and went to wash off the fur Charlie had deposited on his hands.

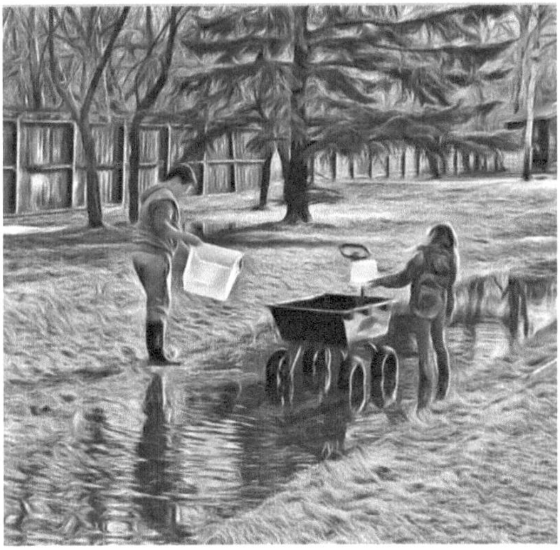

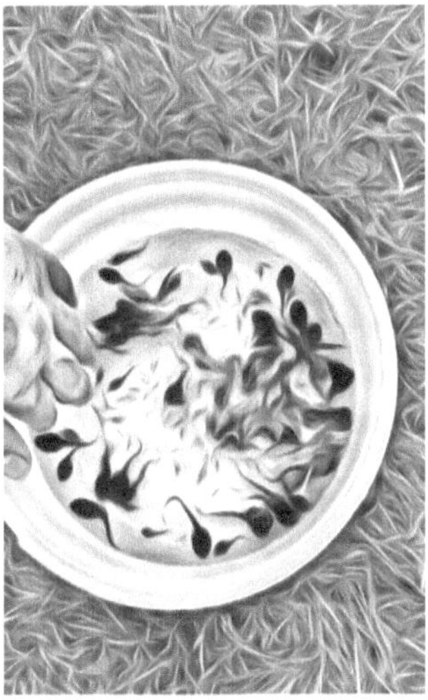

After supper and his shower, Riley and his sister went into the yard to collect frogs and tadpoles. They played in an enormous puddle, and the frogs were enjoying the puddle too. It was like a treasure hunt, finding all those frogs. They scooped tadpoles up and put them into a pail. Once they had over twenty, they set about making a little world for the frogs. They gathered rocks, branches, and grass and put them in the pail with a little bit of water. They enjoyed looking at the frogs and tadpoles. It was super interesting how they all were at different stages of growth and different colours. Some were dark green, and others were bigger and brown. Some of the tadpoles had legs and short tails. Others had long tails and no legs.

Then they set about finding some insects and things to put in their pail for the frogs to munch on. That job was a bit trickier.

"What do frogs eat?" the children asked their parents.

Riley's dad said, "Basically anything small enough to fit into their mouths that also moves across their vision." They went looking for insects that would fit this description.

The family settled down for a fire outside in the forest. It was a crisp fall night, so they were bundled up and came in close around the fire. It was a great way to close the day. Mom had brought out the ingredients for s'mores. Riley jerked his head and blinked his eyes three times, but his family paid no attention. They were all focused on the dancing flames and the sounds of crackling wood in the fire.

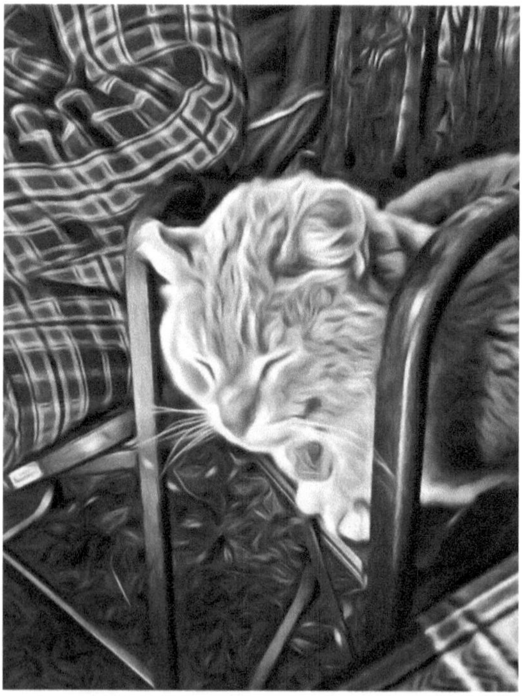

They heard a soft meow, and they all knew that Charlie was on his way over to join them. He weaved between all their legs and got scratches behind his ears. He finally

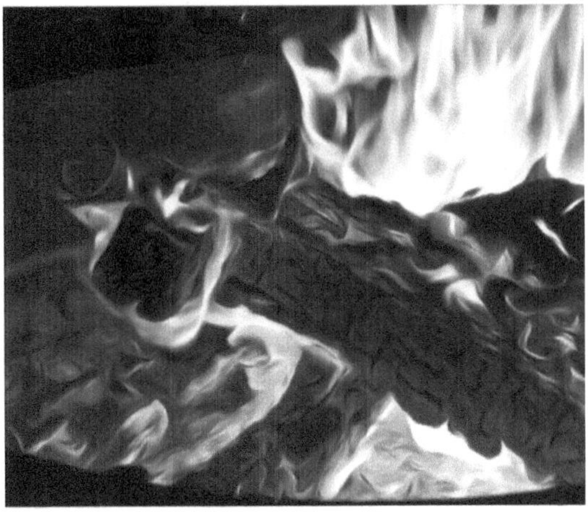

settled on the table beside Riley's mom—the one who is allergic to him, of course. But anyone who knows cats would know that this is what they do, head straight for the person who is allergic to them. Charlie sat on the little table beside her and enjoyed the warmth from the fire.

Riley's arm jerked out and waved in a motion. Then he switched to his gun-shooting tic and made noises to match. It was hard to wait for the marshmallows to roast, so Riley let all his tics out while he watched the marshmallows over the flames. Riley was carefree at that moment and enjoyed the evening so much. Sitting around the fire was one of his favourite things to do. It was even better when they were camping and could just go to bed in the tent when fire time was over.

They batted at a few mosquitoes and Riley said, "Today was a better day, Mom. I think I had a better sleep last night and maybe it helped me. Plus, no assembly in the gym!" They all laughed at this. Both children and Riley's parents couldn't stand assemblies in the gym. It sounded like endless torture, having to sit on the floor! Mom's knees, back, and hips ached at the thought of this. They all laughed at her; the kids called her ancient.

Teasingly, she replied, "I guess that means all the s'mores are for me, since I am the one who is cooking them! Parent tax on the s'mores!" she called out.

Riley's sister wandered off to check on the frogs and found them all still in the pail. She was sad because she knew it was almost bedtime and the frogs would have to be set free. They were so fun to watch. It was amazing to see them climbing the side of the pail with their sticky feet. But her hands were just as sticky as she finished off her s'more. Plus, her mouth and hair also had melted marshmallow strings on them.

The day was coming to a close, and Riley was thankful. His mind was tired with all that had happened in the day. With his body still ticking away, he managed to squeeze in a hug for Charlie and a few more pets. Then they all went in to get ready for bed.

www.ingramcontent.com/pod-product-compliance
Lightning Source LLC
Chambersburg PA
CBHW050342290526
45785CB00006B/2600
* 9 7 8 1 0 3 9 1 9 7 3 2 9 *